The

Golfer's Caddie

A logbook to record information
on everything concerning your
Golfing Game

Golfers...

This small carry it along while you play log book is a great place to keep track of your scores, how well you and your friends played and all the other things you would like to record.

Such as what the course was like and the weather that special day. Little things you want to remember.

Good luck with your golf games, trips, tournaments, and vacations.

And as the PGA says, "Here's to Life under Par!"

Sue Viders
sueviders@comcast.net

Copyright © 2018 Sue Viders
The Golfer's Caddie
ISBN 978-0-942011-72 - 2

Table of Contents

1 - Events

Besides simply playing a round or two of golf with friends and family, it's also fun to play against others.

However, keeping track of these events, especially the sign-up dates if you play in more than one event, makes it necessary to write these dates down.

Plus you probably want to keep track of how you played.

And lastly, one page is for listing other events you might be interested in.

- upcoming tournaments - sign-up dates

- tournaments played in and scores

- list of other events

Events

Upcoming tournaments - sign-up dates

January

Event_____ Location_____

Website_____

Dates_____ Registration date_____

Format_____

Possible partner/partners_____

_____

February

Event_____ Location_____

Website_____

Dates_____ Registration date_____

Format_____

Possible partner/partners_____

_____

Events

Upcoming tournaments - sign-up dates

March

Event_____ Location_____

Website_____

Dates_____ Registration date_____

Format_____

Possible partner/partners_____

_____

April

Event_____ Location_____

Website_____

Dates_____ Registration date_____

Format_____

Possible partner/partners_____

_____

Events

Upcoming tournaments - sign-up dates

May

Event_____ Location_____

Website_____

Dates_____ Registration date_____

Format_____

Possible partner/partners_____

_____

June

Event_____ Location_____

Website_____

Dates_____ Registration date_____

Format_____

Possible partner/partners_____

_____

Events

Upcoming tournaments - sign-up dates

July

Event_____ Location_____

Website_____

Dates_____ Registration date_____

Format_____

Possible partner/partners_____

_____

August

Event_____ Location_____

Website_____

Dates_____ Registration date_____

Format_____

Possible partner/partners_____

_____

Events

Upcoming tournaments - sign-up dates

September

Event_____ Location_____

Website_____

Dates_____ Registration date_____

Format_____

Possible partner/partners_____

_____

October

Event_____ Location_____

Website_____

Dates_____ Registration date_____

Format_____

Possible partner/partners_____

_____

Events

Upcoming tournaments - sign-up dates

November

Event_____ Location_____

Website_____

Dates_____ Registration date_____

Format_____

Possible partner/partners_____

_____

December

Event_____ Location_____

Website_____

Dates_____ Registration date_____

Format_____

Possible partner/partners_____

_____

Events

Tournaments played in and scores

Tournament _____Date_____

    Score_____ Played with_____

    Notes _____

Tournament _____Date_____

    Score_____ Played with_____

    Notes _____

Tournament _____Date_____

    Score_____ Played with_____

    Notes _____

Tournament _____Date_____

    Score_____ Played with_____

    Notes _____

Events

Tournaments played in and scores

Tournament _____Date_____

   Score_____ Played with_____

   Notes _____

Tournament _____Date_____

   Score_____ Played with_____

   Notes _____

Tournament _____Date_____

   Score_____ Played with_____

   Notes _____

Tournament _____Date_____

   Score_____ Played with_____

   Notes _____

Events

List of other events

- _____
_____

- _____
_____

- _____
_____

- _____
_____

- _____
_____

- _____
_____

- _____
_____

- _____
_____

2 - Equipment & Performances

It's interesting to compare your equipment and their performances against those of other players.

So following are a few charts with room for you to record your performance.

Also there is a place to list your favorite golfing equipment brands and the stores where they can be found.

- average hitting distances

- other equipment

- best places to buy golfing stuff

Equipment & Performances

Average hitting distances

	Men	Women	Me	Low	High
Driver	230 yds	200 yds	_____	_____	_____
3-wood	210	180	_____	_____	_____
2-iron	190	170	_____	_____	_____
3-iron	180	160	_____	_____	_____
4-iron	170	150	_____	_____	_____
5-iron	160	140	_____	_____	_____
6-iron	150	130	_____	_____	_____
7-iron	140	120	_____	_____	_____
8-iron	130	110	_____	_____	_____
9-iron	120	100	_____	_____	_____
PW	110	90	_____	_____	_____
SW	90	80	_____	_____	_____
LW	65	55	_____	_____	_____

Equipment & Performances

Other equipment

Bag_____

_____

Shoes_____

_____

Gloves_____

Sunglasses_____ _____

Hats_____

_____

Jackets/rain gear_____

_____

Slacks/shorts/shirts_____

_____

Other stuff

  balls_____

  grips_____

Equipment & Performances

Best places to buy golfing stuff

- _____

_____

- _____

_____

- _____

_____

- _____

_____

- _____

_____

- _____

_____

- _____

_____

3 - Resources

Instruction has come a long way from simply a one on one coach at the country club to golf places where you can practice to your heart's content or where you can follow the online instructors as they show you how it's done.

However, as you know, not all instructors or instructions are right for you and your swing. So as experience teaches us, try a variety of people, places, and U-tube videos and tutorials until you find those personalities that you like and can actually help you with your game.

And hopefully in your area there is a golf place where you can go to work on your drills during the off seasons or when it's raining or snowing.

- instructors

- lessons learned

- miscellaneous

Resources

Instructors

Instructors/coaches you have worked with

Name _____

    Email/phone_____

    Helpful/not helpful_____

    Personality_____

Name _____

    Email/phone_____

    Helpful/not helpful_____

    Personality_____

Name _____

    Email/phone_____

    Helpful/not helpful_____

    Personality_____

Resources

Lessons learned

Drills that are most helpful

_____

_____

_____

_____

What do I need to work on next

_____

_____

_____

_____

Who can best help me

_____

_____

_____

_____

Resources

Miscellaneous

Which golf shops give lessons

_____

_____

_____

Which clubs have a pro that gives great lessons

_____

_____

_____

Which sites give the best tutorials

_____

_____

_____

Which friend can and does help me the most

_____

_____

_____

4 - Golf Courses

They are everywhere from city municipal courses to the local country clubs to the courses all over the world.

Some courses are fairly easy, while others are extremely difficult. Some courses overlook the ocean, some the deserts while others are high in the mountains.

It's fun to keep track of which courses you have played, the weather, the day you played, and, of course, who you played with and how well you did.

- local

- USA

- international

Golf Courses

Local

Name and location_____

    website_____ date _____

    level of difficulty/9 or 18 holes_____

    fees and reservation policies_____

    weather conditions_____

    person(s) played with_____

    how well did I play (score)_____

    notes_____

Name and location_____

    website_____ date _____

    level of difficulty/9 or 18 holes_____

    fees and reservation policies_____

    weather conditions_____

    person(s) played with_____

    how well did I play (score)_____

    notes_____

Golf courses

USA

Name and location_____

website_____ date _____

level of difficulty/9 or 18 holes_____

fees and reservation policies_____

weather conditions_____

person(s) played with_____

how well did I play (score)_____

notes_____

Name and location_____

website_____ date _____

level of difficulty/9 or 18 holes_____

fees and reservation policies_____

weather conditions_____

person(s) played with_____

how well did I play (score)_____

notes_____

Golf Courses

International

Name and location_____

    website_____ date _____

    level of difficulty/9 or 18 holes_____

    fees and reservation policies_____

    weather conditions_____

    person(s) played with_____

    how well did I play (score)_____

    notes_____

Name and location_____

    website_____ date _____

    level of difficulty/9 or 18 holes_____

    fees and reservation policies_____

    weather conditions_____

    person(s) played with_____

    how well did I play (score)_____

    notes_____

5 - Golf Resorts

Whether it's a vacation or simply your favorite place to play, it behooves you to check out certain aspects before embarking on the trip.

Time of year, discount packages, and senior offerings can save you tons, well, not tons, but a substantial amount of money.

Be sure, however, to check each place out individually as packages vary greatly, not only in price but what they provide, while some vacation destinations leave all that free time up to you to solve.

- favorite places

- vacation destinations

- golf vacation packages

Golf Resorts

Favorite places

Name and location_____

   website_____

   courses_____

   cost_____ discounts available_____

   amenities included_____

   lessons available_____

   side trips available_____

   notes_____

Name and location_____

   website_____

   courses_____

   cost_____ discounts available_____

   amenities included_____

   lessons available_____

   side trips available_____

   notes_____

Golf Resorts

Vacation destinations

Name and location_____

website_____

courses_____

cost_____ discounts available_____

amenities included_____

lessons available_____

side trips available_____

notes_____

Name and location_____

website_____

courses_____

cost_____ discounts available_____

amenities included_____

lessons available_____

side trips available_____

notes_____

Golf Resorts

Golf vacation packages

Name and location_____

    website_____

    courses_____

    cost_____ discounts available_____

    amenities included_____

    lessons available_____

    side trips available_____

    notes_____

Name and location_____

    website_____

    courses_____

    cost_____ discounts available_____

    amenities included_____

    lessons available_____

    side trips available_____

    notes_____

6 - Scores

Golf is one of those wonderful games that prays constantly on the players ego, which is okay, but because of our egos we need to talk about our scores, our great hits and, of course, those tricky sand saves.

If you don't know your "true" handicap numbers, have an instructor or pro show you how to figure it out. It will really help you with all your scores in the future.

Knowing your handicap will enable you to play with other players whose skill level (handicap) is the same or nearly the same as yours. This way the game is much more fun and challenging.

- handicap history

- highlights from rounds

- score cards to cherish

Scores

Handicap history

Record how your handicap has changed

My first handicap was _____

    year_____ at what course/golf club_____

    and the scores were_____

My next handicap was _____

    year_____ at what course/golf club_____

    and the scores were_____

And now my handicap is _____

    year_____ at what course/golf club_____

    and the scores were_____

But, my goal for my next handicap is_____

_____

Scores

Highlights

Course_____ Date_____

Score_____

Handicap_____

Number of fairways hits_____

Number of greens hits_____

Number of putts_____

Sand shots _____

Eagles (which holes) _____

Birdies (which holes)_____

Par (which holes)_____

Bogeys (which holes)_____

Other interesting shots_____

_____

_____

_____

_____

Scores

Score cards to cherish

There are several ways to save your best score cards:

1 - put them in an envelope at the back of this book_____

_____

2 - arrange them artistically and have them framed_____

_____

3 - hang them on a wall where you can see them_____

_____

4 - put score on license plate_____

_____

‒

5 - if you play a lot of cards, have a card set made_____

_____

6 - other ideas_____

_____

_____

_____

7 - Horn Tooting

There is a saying that nicely fits your best shots…

"If you don't toot your own horn, don't complain if there's no music."

Of course, don't get carried away. No one likes a bragger. But if you don't say something about your great shots, your ego will definitely suffer.

To keep these great achievements from getting out of hand, sometimes a physical reminder is needed.

How about a nice glass golf ball crystal for your desk at work or a plaque on the wall? And for your golfing buddies, perhaps get them each a t-shirt with "hole-in-one by (your name here)" written on it. Subtle, right?

- hole in one

- shots to remember

- shots to forget

Horn Tooting

Hole in one

When and where did this happen:

year and course _____

what hole_____

club used_____

distance_____

witnesses_____

_____

When and where did this happen:

year and course _____

what hole_____

club used_____

distance_____

witnesses_____

_____

Horn Tooting

Shots to remember

What other shots are you extremely proud of?

number of fairways hits

_____

_____

greens in regulation

_____

_____

number of putts

_____

_____

sand saves

_____

_____

other

_____

_____

_____

_____

Horn Tooting

Shots to forget

Now, how about those lousy shots you can never forget

number of fairway shots missed

_____

_____

number of greens shots missed

_____

_____

number of close putts missed

_____

_____

sand shots you couldn't make

_____

_____

other mess-ups shots

_____

_____

_____

_____

_____

_____

8 - Organizations/Clubs

There are a jillion different types of golfing organizations, clubs, businesses and specialized groups. And even if there weren't any, you and your friends could form your own.

Why bother to belong to a group? Because socialization is the second most wonderful gift golf gives to you after the first most wonderful gift, which is exercise.

Following is a list of some of the groups you might want to consider joining.

- local/country club groups

- specialized groups

- national organizations

Organizations/Clubs

Local/country club groups

Local groups

Name_____

   website _____

   purpose of the group_____

   leaders name, phone, and email address_____

   _____

   what I can do for the group_____

   _____

Name_____

   website _____

   purpose of the group_____

   leaders name, phone, and email address_____

   _____

   what I can do for the group_____

   _____

Organizations/Clubs

Specialized groups

List those groups that give tournaments for charity:

Name_____

   website _____

   purpose of the group_____

   leaders name, phone, and email address_____

   _____

   what I can do for the group_____

   _____

Name_____

   website _____

   purpose of the group_____

   leaders name, phone, and email address_____

   _____

   what I can do for the group_____

   _____

Organizations/Clubs

National organizations

Name_____

website _____

purpose of the group_____

leaders name, phone, and email address_____

_____

what I can do for the group_____

_____

Name_____

website _____

purpose of the group_____

leaders name, phone, and email address_____

_____

what I can do for the group_____

_____

9 - Golfing Buddies

Ah, those wonderful friends that also love golf and love to play whenever they can.

Following is a place to save their names, phone and email addresses along with notes on their level of skill and times available.

- contact information

Golfing Buddies

Contact information

Name_____

phone and email_____

address_____

skill level_____

availability_____

best days and times to play_____

notes_____

_____

Name_____

phone and email_____

address_____

skill level_____

availability_____

best days and times to play_____

notes_____

_____

Golfing Buddies

Contact information

Name_____

phone and email_____

address_____

skill level_____

availability_____

best days and times to play_____

notes_____

_____

Name_____

phone and email_____

address_____

skill level_____

availability_____

best days and times to play_____

notes_____

_____

Golfing Buddies

Contact information

Name_____

   phone and email_____

   address_____

   skill level_____

   availability_____

   best days and times to play_____

   notes_____

_____

Name_____

   phone and email_____

   address_____

   skill level_____

   availability_____

   best days and times to play_____

   notes_____

_____

Golfing Buddies

Contact information

Name_____

phone and email_____

address_____

skill level_____

availability_____

best days and times to play_____

notes_____

_____

Name_____

phone and email_____

address_____

skill level_____

availability_____

best days and times to play_____

notes_____

_____

Golfing Buddies

Contact information

Name_____

    phone and email_____

    address_____

    skill level_____

    availability_____

    best days and times to play_____

    notes_____

_____

Name_____

    phone and email_____

    address_____

    skill level_____

    availability_____

    best days and times to play_____

    notes_____

_____

Notes

Notes

www.ingramcontent.com/pod-product-compliance
Lightning Source LLC
Chambersburg PA
CBHW060524280326
41933CB00014B/3099